CLEAN BEAUTY FOR THE MIND

Three Ways to Cleanse Toxic Words of Others

By

Karlene Markham

*"**Let go of your past, transform your thoughts, and embrace the life you were designed to live.** The words in the book, Clean Beauty for the Mind, draw me in like I am sitting and having coffee with the author. They open my heart to know and understand her, providing insight on how her story can help me process and grow in mine. Karlene Markham encourages her readers to go deeper, past the search for surface beauty, into the hidden places where toxic words may have caused damage to our hearts and souls.*

I have read a lot on this topic but have not read something that gives these clear steps and a way to help first filter and then process past, present, and future experiences with words.

Drawing on personal experience and wisdom, Karlene provides practical insight in how to evaluate and deal with words that are spoken over us. In sharing this insight, Karlene allows us a glimpse into her own heart and the way she has protected her ability to live with intentionality, provide life-giving words to those around her, and reflect the true beauty that radiates and shines out of every area of her life.

Clean Beauty for the Mind will equip you with practical steps to let go of the past, transform your thoughts, and reach forward to embrace the life you were designed to live."

- Donna Jo Hewitt, Elementary School Teacher & Vice Principal

*"**A must read!** I read this book in two short evenings - yet it's impactful information will stay with me for a lifetime! Karlene shares a personal experience and the important lesson she learned by going through it, then explains three powerful ways to block out negative words of others. I loved this book so much and can't wait for future releases by this insightful author!"*

- Laurie Snure, Editor, *The Jewels of Fate Series*

- Paperback ISBN# 979-8849621029
- eBook ISBN# B0BBTMXL6F

Author Photograph by Bill Markham
Cover Image by Karlene Markham

⇒ Instagram: #cleanbeautyforthemind
⇒ Facebook: @cleanbeautyforthemind

www.cleanbeautyforthemind.com

DEDICATION

This book is dedicated to my cherished family.

To my inspiring parents, my first models who live out what it looks like to use the power of words for good in this world to this day.

To my wonderful husband, who consistently uses his words to encourage me to go for it in life, no matter what. And to my amazing children and new grandbaby, who inspire me daily to want to use my own words to be the best mom (and mormor) I can be.

There are some things we tend to take for granted in life. My family is not one of those things. I'm beyond grateful for the gifts that they are.

That is, and always will be, priceless.

TABLE OF CONTENTS

Introduction 8

Chapter One: The Announcement -
          When Words Leave You Speechless 12

Chapter Two: The Affront - The Gift That Kept on Giving 14

Chapter Three: Uninvited 16

Chapter Four: Raw Awakening 18
       Part 1: Practice Doesn't Make Perfect 18
       Part 2: A Little Less Limbo, Please 20
       Part 3: Re-writing Your Story 22

Chapter Five: The Three Filters - That Clarified My Thoughts 26
       Part 1: Intentional Clarity 26
       Part 2: Setting Up a Standard 27
       Part 3: The Three Filtering Questions 30
          A. Filter #1 30
          B. Filter #2 31
          C. Filter #3 32

Chapter Six: We All Stand for Something 36

Chapter Seven: No Apology? No Issue. 38
       Part 1: Entitlement Weakens Us 38
       Part 2: Forgiveness Makes Us Stronger 39

Chapter Eight: Hope is Ahead 44

Concluding Thoughts 46

Bibliography 50

Acknowledgements 52

About the Author 54

INTRODUCTION

If you've picked up this book, I'm betting you're also a fan of the 'clean beauty' genre. Whether you've begun tackling the tiny print on labels or are just becoming aware, you've likely got some conscious perception of the popular expression.

Until recently, I don't know if I'd stopped to delve into what a true definition of clean beauty would even look like.

Is it just an absence of toxins?

Or is it something a little more profound?

When it comes to 'beauty,' too often, it's the outward version that's been the celebrated focus of humanity. No matter the gender, the external allure often receives most of the gold stars, the loudest shouts, and the highest accolades.

We've become so hard on ourselves, comparing with others, based on the outward alone. So, we've settled for a status quo of merely one facet of beauty when *so many more forms are to be celebrated!*

Many people who leave an influential mark on the world have done so because of how they stewarded their minds and hearts.

Consider Martin Luther King Junior. We admire him for how he inspired others by sharing those powerful words, "*I Have a Dream...*" while leading a civil rights movement that focused on nonviolent protest. His vision of equality and civil disobedience changed the world for his children and the children of all oppressed people.

Or take Mother Teresa who helped Calcutta's poor, sick, and needy people. In her lifetime, she helped create 623 missions in 123 countries. This was achieved starting with her influential words, which she simply, yet effectively, lived out in action.

Both public figures are extreme examples, but I reference them to illustrate the reality of what is possible when we 'live clean,' inside-out.

To be clear, I don't pretend to be a trained therapist when it comes to advising. During a brief dabble in a college counseling class, I quickly realized that with so many layers embedded in that broad field, that wasn't going to be my aim.

At the same time, the spark to want to help others move forward has always lingered inside me.

I just wanted to do it a little differently.

My passion for helping others see a release from negative words that hold us back has been growing within me for years, as I've seen firsthand what can happen.

But now, I feel a greater sense of urgency to have this conversation. With recent events, society has been hit hard with a tsunami of toxic words and thoughts. In its wake, we now have an incredible opportunity to become more intentional and aware of our outlook.

That's why I'm even more grateful for the timing of this opportunity to share this with you today. Maybe you want to move forward, or perhaps you're just curious to know more first.

There is incredible worth found in our real-life experiences. I've realized that immense value is created when we compound our experiences, both personally and with others.

So, I thought, *what if I took a risk, put on some vulnerability, and opened up about some of my own journeys, with the hope that maybe others could be helped too?*

My friend, the words you're about to read reflect that answer – from my heart to yours. Wherever you're at on your quest, 'Clean Beauty for the Mind' can be your muster point toward a beautiful life.

Together, we'll explore powerful ways to set up a new 'thought standard' to remove the grit from negative words that too easily fill our minds.

And that simple action has the potential to affect your entire future.

So, if you feel you've been left floundering in the wake of too much heaviness after being on the receiving end of negative words, this is for you. If you're tired of being chained to limited thinking and are ready for a fresh perspective at last, then, my friend, this is your time.

May your heart be lifted as you read!

CHAPTER ONE: THE ANNOUNCEMENT
When Words Leave You Speechless

I was elated, exhausted, and feeling incredibly vulnerable as I lay regaining my strength in the maternity ward. The birthing experience had been profoundly challenging, but recovery was progressing well. It was a beautiful afternoon, and I was a pretty fresh first-time Momma.

My hospital stay was interrupted by a gift.

After going through a life-changing event like none other, anticipation filled my heart as to who the thoughtful gift-giver might be. Undoubtedly, it must be a congratulatory message or token of some sort to mark this joyous occasion!

I opened up my heart to receive the gift.

Loosening the envelope's seal, I was eager to read the card to discover who the considerate sender might be. I mean, a gift delivered right to my hospital room?

Of course, that was an even bigger deal, as it usually meant it must be from an extra special person! But, as I began to read the words, I was stunned. In fact, I had to do a double-take and read it a second time to take it in properly.

The most toxic words ever spoken to me filled both pages of the card, words rife with derisive insults, slander, and sheer hatred.

The intent was impossible to miss.

In the face of this verbal attack, my vulnerability quickly rose to the surface. A shockwave of infinite confusion and sadness echoed.

I mean, how could anyone DO something like this? And why now, at one of the happiest moments in my life?

I had a crucial choice: would I allow those words to inflict their intended wounds or not?

Numbly, I handed the card to my husband. Quickly scanning the words, he instantly made the right choice – he threw it away.

With the onset of a new Momma's emotions hitting hard, the blunt force of these words was almost too much to bear. As I lay in that hospital bed, that personal attack on my very character and reputation felt magnified.

But there was more.

CHAPTER TWO: THE AFFRONT
The Gift That Kept on Giving

I couldn't have known it yet, but I was about to discover an equally venomous gift that accompanied those toxic words. Still in its unwrapped state, a gift customarily associated with an act of kindness was to be a poison-tipped arrow.

Not long afterward, in the whirlwind of excitement in bringing our sweet newborn home from the hospital, my mind somehow managed to hit pause on what had just happened. For the time being, the joy of welcoming our tiny babe home momentarily overshadowed earlier events.

Perhaps it was curiosity, or maybe I still wanted to believe the best about this situation. I don't know. But at last, I chose to open the unwrapped gift. The contents were what I'd call a most unusual celebratory gift: two jars of preserved beans.

It turned out the present was a perfect pairing with the card. The painful reality stung hard: the contents of those jars were entirely rotten. And since spoiled preserves can lead to botulism, even death, they too immediately met with the same fate as the toxic card.

Could this really be happening, or was this some kind of bad dream?

Did the sender seriously not realize that rotten preserves could have dangerously harmed my sweet baby as well?

CHAPTER THREE: UNINVITED

Hopefully, a situation like this has never happened to you. It's so astonishing that sometimes when I think back, I want to shake my head in disbelief at the events.

Maybe what you've read so far has already begun triggering familiar emotions. Perhaps another circumstance is even now coming to mind, and it's painful. Pay attention to it – your thoughts are on alert for a reason.

That day in the hospital, the uninvited seeds of self-doubt had been thrust into my freshly wounded heart.

Although I'd never wish something like this on anyone, that event would eventually serve a purpose in my life in days to come.

Fast forward to the wonder of two more beautifully incredible babies – my arms and heart were so full that the seemingly distant event had gotten a little lost in the recesses of my mind for a time. However, I'd never processed that earlier gifting incident properly.

Even though the sender had personalized the message, boldly signing the card, removing all doubt as to who it was from, I hadn't attempted to seek that person out to at least talk. Racking my brain, I couldn't think of anything that might have happened to spur those words on from the sender. Even from the little I knew of the person; such callousness seemed inconceivable.

Sadly, I was probably more concerned with offending the individual rather than risking a confrontation – or even standing up for myself.

Deep down, I'd hoped simply ignoring the situation would eventually make it just go away.

But that's not what happened. Just because you're able to dismiss words temporarily through distraction doesn't mean they cease to exist in your mind.

Although repressed, those words hovered within my subliminal thoughts in years to come, even to the point where they'd impact the way I'd make some decisions. The seeds of self-doubt had begun to grow, affecting my openness to being known by others.

I mean, what if there was even the slightest hint of truth in those words? Would people really want to be associated with someone like me?

Would the risk be worth it?

CHAPTER FOUR: RAW AWAKENING

I can't pinpoint the exact day when my awareness finally began to surface. But thankfully, over time, a greater perception emerged within.

For too long, precious energy had been wasted fighting against the invisible stigma of untrustworthy words. The effect had compounded over time through inevitable moments of further negativity.

Let me explain. When we start to believe a set of toxic words about ourselves, even if they seem harmless at first, our resistance slowly gets chipped away over time, even causing our very immunity levels to be compromised.

I'd have opportunities yet hold myself back, believing others might also echo those words I never wanted to hear again. So often, it became easier to just avoid possibilities than to take risks.

PART 1: Practice Doesn't Make Perfect

It wasn't as though every minute of every day was impacted. But over time, it soon became evident that a pattern was forming. Proof of that was shown in too many missed moments and situations I'd stepped aside from embracing.

When new thought patterns form, it means our brain creates pathways. 'Myelin Sheaths' form in our brains to insulate nerve cells and form 'superhighways' that allow for more efficient pathways through which electrical messages are carried. The more we think of or do something, the stronger these highways become. [1]

Maybe you can identify. Possibly you've begun to notice a pattern too, but just aren't sure what to do about it. You may even feel an unexplained sense that your heart is weighed down; something is 'off,' but you're not sure why.

Or maybe you know exactly why – you feel the heaviness of antagonistic words, but you're at a loss. As a result, you're feeling immobilized from moving forward.

Stay with me here. I want to offer help today.

Because I hadn't properly dealt with those words right away, the soundtrack of my mind was on repeat, playing negative lyrics over and over, adding the latest dissonant words as time went on.

Sounds harmless, right?

Our minds are hardwired to be efficient, with powerful potential to improve whatever we focus on. So, in the case of practicing or repeating negative thought patterns, we'll just get better and better at it.

Here's what happens behind the scenes when we keep the negative track on repeat: the injurious thoughts gain in intensity, becoming more significant than they were in the first place. They gain in volume, becoming louder, drowning out our ability to better hear or express good words we want to give and receive each new day. They also gain in momentum, picking up speed. When all this collides, we have even quicker, more efficient access to that harmful memory associated with the original event.

Every single moment we reserve space for those thoughts, it's a decision to go in reverse. Suddenly we're back in the past, feeling 'all the feels' of those moments, replaying all the words repeatedly. We're even providing the glue to help them 'stick' in our minds.

As a result, we can get really good at living in the past.

PART 2: Less Limbo, Please

Accepting the choice to live in the past is like deciding to diminish the joys of today's moments just waiting to be experienced. In addition, living in past negative thought patterns restricts our creativity for new hopes and plans for the future.

It could even be the most glorious day, with the sun's warmth shining on us. However, we can't appreciate it to its fullest extent because we're marooned under a cloud of negative words from the past.

Over time, an unbroken ripple effect of negative words can create what I call emotional tidal waves inside us. These far-reaching waves can impact us by washing away our confidence. And when our confidence is adversely affected, a lack of trust in our ability to achieve goals simultaneously erodes.

I hope you're beginning to understand the effects of what really happens when we hold on to 'seemingly harmless' negative words.

Had I recognized all this earlier, I could have been directing more valuable spirit and passion into what I believed to be true, rather than wasting significant energy fighting the false.

Because I have walked through it, I want to offer an opportunity to speed up the process, leaving the past behind. I want you to be able to shed destructive words and thoughts that don't serve you.

It became clear that I needed a standard to help distill those past and subsequent negative words.

As I processed, this realization hit me: when something harsh happens during a time of high vulnerability, we can become even more susceptible to adverse effects than we would otherwise be.

Let me say that another way, because the meaning is so worth remembering.

The deeper our level of rawness at the time, the greater the pain from wounds inflicted.

Timing matters.

For a season, I'd found myself stuck in an 'emotional limbo,' a temporary state where there's a lack of movement either forward or backward in life or relationships.

Perhaps this sounds familiar to you. Like you've been here before. And even though your situation will look different, you still reflect on similar emotions. It could be that the words you're reading right now are triggering reminders of toxic words from your past which need to be dealt with. Or maybe you know someone struggling in this area, and you can't stop thinking about how they would benefit from this conversation too.

It's possible you're just breathing a sigh of relief, knowing you're not alone in what you've been walking through.

Whatever your situation, I know this: being in limbo indefinitely is uncomfortable. And left to its natural progression, staying in limbo leads to emotional roadblocks that slow us down in life.

As for me, something needed to change.

But change is not easy — even when it's for the better! Just thinking about it can be a hurdle when we've gotten used to set patterns. If change was easy, people would be running towards it more regularly. However, even being willing to consider it and follow through will set you apart.

Do you ever wonder why it's simpler to think, *I'll take action, but I'll do it tomorrow because I've got way too much going on today!*

Even though we may get a sense of 'buying time' when we delay taking action, it's only a façade, a magician's trick to distract us from what's really happening.

Further, when we put off dealing with something, there's no gain. Even worse, we're only losing valuable time and opportunities. By procrastinating, we're robbing our future of potentially unforgettable moments yet to be lived.

PART 3: Re-writing Your Story

So, what about you? What's your story?

No matter our starting point, I know the future can look different when we first revise our internal story: *that's the story we tell ourselves about ourselves.* And every great story has its main characters.

Donald Miller, author of *Hero on a Mission*, unpacks the four main characters in great detail. He states, "*If we play the victim, we're doomed to fail. A villain will not create genuine bonds. But if we play the hero or the guide, our lives will flourish.*"[2]

If you're familiar with this, have you ever stopped to consider which role you'd relate to most in your life story? Is it the hero, the guide, the victim, or the villain?

If this feels brand-new for you, what's your first thought that comes to mind?

We've all been victims at some time – it's a natural part of being human. Situations beyond our control can happen. Maybe people don't treat or speak to us with dignity or care.

That's not the kind of victim we're talking about here.

Instead, I'm referring to becoming a 'chronic victim' where something has happened to us, and we keep rehearsing it in our minds. Rather than moving forward from it, we remain in that victim mindset – *long after the event has passed.*

The crazy thing is, it's so easy to play the victim in our story without intending to – or realizing it.

So how can we tell if we're acting like the victim?

Please, do NOT feel discouraged if you see yourself in any of the indicators I'm about to list. Becoming self-aware is a positive thing.

Remember, we've ALL felt these ways at one time or another. The beauty is when we have that realization; it's a great gift – it means now we're in a position to do something to alter our future for better days to come!

Here are a few key indicators that you might be feeling like the victim in your story, if: [3]

- *You genuinely feel life is against you.*
- *You blame others for the way life is.*
- *You feel powerless to change.*
- *You feel attacked when someone tries to offer helpful feedback.*
- *Feeling bad about yourself brings you pleasure.*
- *You attract people who blame others and complain about their life.*

For me, I was done with any part of being a victim in my mind.

In your internal story (the story you tell yourself about yourself), I want you to be able to feel you're one of the characters who flourish. In so doing, I know you can feel more alive and become one who helps others have a new perspective in life too!

But this new story cannot be rewritten without action on our part.

Get ready. Because in this next chapter, we're going to reveal some powerful tools that have the potential to help you change the way you look at toxic words – for good.

KEY CHAPTER TAKEAWAYS:

Many people can go a whole lifetime without ever having their own 'raw awakening' or awareness. Although it's not an easy realization to have, it plays an important role in whether or not we'll grow from there.

- **Practice Doesn't Make Perfect** – The more we 'practice' or rehearse negative words, the more deeply ingrained they'll become into our thoughts. The unbroken ripple-effects of negative words can impact us by washing away our confidence. When that's adversely affected, a lack of trust in our ability to achieve goals can erode as well.

- **Less Limbo, Please** – Being stuck in 'emotional limbo' not only hurts us, but can also hurt our most cherished relationships. When we stay in 'limbo,' we're robbing our own future of the amazing potential that's ahead.

- **Re-writing Your Story** – Each of our stories has four main characters: the hero, the guide, the victim, or the villain. The things we tell ourselves about ourselves will likely get lived out in our life stories.

- **Key Indicators** – With realization comes opportunity for decision.

CHAPTER FIVE: THE THREE FILTERS
That Clarified My Thoughts

PART 1: Intentional Clarity

I'd finally realized the need to establish a better way to deal with past words over me, to better safeguard the future for myself, my family, and so many I care deeply about.

I wanted my cherished children to have the healthiest version possible of their mom. And since kids learn so much about confidence from what's being modeled, being an influence for good mattered to me even more.

In my mind, if I could work on becoming the person I'd want to be in relationship with, too, that would be a worthy goal to pursue.

When you have your 'raw awakening,' it can change the trajectory not only of your future but also that of your family and many others you influence.

Even if you don't think you have any impact on others, you do. Consider how you make others feel after you've been with them. That's influence!

One way to help develop clarity here, is to ask:

- *"What am I modeling for those around me?"*
- *"Am I the kind of person I'd like to be in relationship with?"*

When our mindset is in a better place, we can do so much good for others and the world around us.

When thinking about negative emotions that remain after others' words, our first impulse can often be to bury them. If we suppress them deeply enough, they might even disappear from our thoughts – for a while.

But what if being aware of those negative emotions actually helps us?

Surprisingly, negative emotions play a valuable role in our lives too. They shine a light on what's going on inside of us. In fact, we can't grow unless we experience some adversity. And when I think about when I've learned the most, it's been through more challenging seasons.

Don't get me wrong – it's not like I want to repeat those difficult seasons. But it's in these times when I've gained new perspectives I wouldn't otherwise have.

An awareness of those emotions can propel us to finally deal with what's happening. We can harness how we feel during sadness, fear, or anxiety and use those times as a powerful springboard to propel us forward.

That happened in my life: a sense of clarity finally came into view. At last, I was finished letting even a corner of my mind be adversely impacted. Armed with a new understanding, I intuitively sought a connection point I could stand behind.

PART 2: Setting Up a Standard

Because I love visuals, I needed to first find an analogy that resonated with me – and I needed to own it.

I was drawn to the visual of a water filter because it so perfectly clarifies the intent here. Using a filter allows access to clean water, free of pollutants, making it healthier and taste better too. In fact, without filters, we can quickly become sick from contamination. (The parallels we can draw in life here are so good!)

Next, I needed to decide where I wanted to see myself in the future.

We don't need to be rocket scientists to know the success of reaching our destination on any road trip is determined by the map we use. If we don't know where we want to be, it's tough to know where to begin.

Many of us wander through life, just letting things happen – not being intentional about where we really want to go. Unfortunately, it's easy to get caught in that mindset and settle.

Consider this, though. Perhaps we lose some of that purpose because we've listened to the voices of those who did not have our best in mind. And maybe we've given those voices permission to impact us without realizing it.

There's also a massive matter of confusion. With so many decisions in life, it's way too easy to get overwhelmed and not know where to start. In fact, a confused mind will always say no. This is why knowing where to begin is valuable. That's when clarity begins: a chance to say "_yes_" to progress.

When it comes to the overwhelm, I've found this statement to be helpful:

Part of figuring out what you DO want in life is determining what you DON'T want.

I've found that the filter I'm about to share is an effective tool for establishing what we DON'T want so we can eliminate that and make room for the good stuff we DO want.

And here's the good stuff that resonated with me: I wanted to become focused on being more life-giving with thoughts, speech, and actions – both towards others and to myself. To live more fully, free of the weight of negative words replaying in my mind that held me back.

So, because this helped me, I'm excited to share my filter with you too.

The filter isn't hype.

Instead, it's a powerful means that can help take you closer to where you want to be today and in the future.

This filter can also be a compelling key to helping unlock chains of negativity that have kept your past thoughts tightly caged.

You may still not be aware of the need to find a proactive way to cleanse those toxic words of others from your mind. So, go ahead and save this tool for a rainy day then, because my friend, it's a guarantee that day will come!

But if you're in a place where you've stopped believing it's even possible to get 'unstuck,' I want to encourage you today with a simple starting point.

As part of creating a new standard of thought, I call this powerful tool my 'emotional filter.'

My emotional filter is made up of three key benchmark questions. When I think about, hear, or read words directed my way, and I'm not totally sure where they belong, there are three 'filtering questions' that help clarify things for me.

These questions I'm about to share will determine how incoming words will get 'strained' from that moment onward.

It may take a little time to stick, but my friend, progress is still progress.

PART 3: The Three Filtering Questions

A. Filter #1: *"Are the words true?"*

If the answer is "no," then I need to disregard them as the impurities they are to avoid thought contamination. And if picturing that visual of a filter is helpful, I'll do that too.

If the answer is "yes," I need to look more closely. When I'm blinded to reality, that doesn't help anyone – least of all me. Nobody benefits if I remain oblivious to areas I need to work on in life. There's no such thing as being 'blissfully unaware' in this context.

If you're a person of faith, exploring the question, *"Who does God say I am?"* can lead to a compelling awareness that can help with the standard of thought. A beautiful montage of words exquisitely crafted in the biblical book of *Psalm 139* expresses how worthy and accepted we are. And when I internalize this, it stays constant because, thankfully, it won't be based just on my merits but on what I believe God's character to be. And in a rapidly adapting world, that's a great source of strength.

Okay, but what about when there's an uncomfortable truth in words spoken about me?

That doesn't mean I'm a terrible person. It's just an opportunity for growth — a chance to become aware, move out of my comfort zone, and begin thriving! The goal of life can't just be to agree with everyone or constantly avoid being uncomfortable.

Far from it!

If that were the case, no achievements would ever be made; no mountains would ever be climbed; no innovations would ever have advanced the world. Perhaps worst of all, though, if we lived our whole lives trying to avoid being uncomfortable, no hearts or relationships would have the opportunity for healing.

Allowing for a "*yes*" response to this question simply means I have work to do. Furthermore, it signifies I now have an opportunity ahead of me.

And saying "*yes*" to growth means I can finally start becoming more of who I am designed to be.

Can you picture the possibilities yet?

B. Filter #2: *"Do I respect, admire, or want to be anything like the person who's spoken these words?"*

If the answer is "no," then I need to choose once again to discard the words as impurities that won't be passing through the filter into my life.

I recognize people don't always stay the same. Maybe we once admired that person, but unfortunately, their character has degraded since that time. Toxic words paired with fractured respect aren't an easy combination.

Using the filter will help clarify this, funneling those words away from your thoughts, keeping the pure, trustworthy, and clean, and purging the rest.

If the answer is "yes," these words will carry more weight. When the person sharing the words is someone I do respect, look up to or want to become more like, the words they speak also mean more to me. Those words hold more intrinsic value because I trust the source.

And trust is a sacred thing.

Holding respect or admiration for someone can be a beautiful thing too, but it should be done with wisdom.

That's why it's good to ask yourself *"why you admire the person?"*

- *Is it for reasons that support your core values?*
- *Are they 'others-focused' or 'self-focused?'*
- *If you really aspire to be like them, what about this person draws you?*

The more you respect, admire, or want to be like someone, the more heavily invested you also allow your emotions to become as well.

So many times, this is a wonderful place to be. However, we still need to be aware that we don't give another person's opinion too much sway over us. Balance is important.

You can see the value of having a standard of thought. A target to aim for helps better understand who to trust.

Trust is earned over time, as I've seen the person's character, witnessed them in action, and found that their words also align with their lives.

In other words, I can believe in the behavior of the person speaking these words.

C. Filter #3: *"What can I learn from these words?"*

The answer to this filtering question is never "*nothing*." It can't be. As long as I have a pulse, I've got things to learn through positive or negative experiences. When we welcome growth, however challenging, we can be continually spurred on to live more of our potential.

Answering this filtering question is also a fantastic opportunity to become more self-aware. I don't want to be gullible, thinking everyone else is at fault, never taking personal responsibility for the situation. But, at the same time, neither will I settle for believing I'm a victim. If we approach the situation with humility, that can go a long way to making life more fulfilling.

When someone speaks unfeeling, untrue, or even inflammatory words, we always have choices in responding. If we fire back with equally toxic words, we merely escalate the situation. Hurling incendiary words right back is like pouring gas on a bonfire. When the conversation is over, the embers of destruction are all that remain.

But if we genuinely seek clarity in conversation, a powerful place to start is simply by asking questions. Many ask questions but aren't really looking to hear an answer. This becomes evident quickly.

However, if we ask questions to understand, that can change the outcome altogether.

When we speak the truth confidently while avoiding the bait of sinking into retorts of lethal depths, we hold the key to opening the door to our potential.

KEY CHAPTER TAKEAWAYS:

- **Intentional Clarity** – Even when we don't recognize it, each of our lives impact others in some way! One way to help develop clarity here, is to ask:

    o   *"What am I modeling for those around me?"*

    o   *"Am I the kind of person I'd like to be in relationship with?"*

- **Setting Up a Standard** – Establishing values will help us with setting up a standard of thought. Defining who we're wanting to become, why we're aiming for that, what that looks like, and a plan to get there is vital.

- **Three Filtering Questions** – Ask yourself:

    ⇒ **#1:** *Are the words true?*

    ⇒ **#2:** *Do I respect, admire, or want to be anything like the person who's spoken those words?*

    ⇒ **#3:** *What can I learn from these words?*

CHAPTER SIX: WE ALL STAND FOR SOMETHING

It's more significant to be known for what we stand for rather than just what we fight against.

Have you ever noticed how much easier it is to lean into the negative first?

Think about it: if you spontaneously asked three people today what they were 'against,' you'd probably have three very instant responses.

But then if you asked those same three people what they were 'for,' they'd probably have a more challenging time responding as eagerly.

Why is that?

Spending all our energy on what we're against is the low-hanging fruit in life. It's the easiest way to live. Of course, anyone can live that way, but it doesn't lead to helpful places.

It takes much more effort to 'mine gold' and seek the good. And when we find it, focusing on the good helps us feel better simultaneously.

It's true – no two situations in life are the same. There's no way I can know your journey like you do! We all have unique challenges.

No matter our situation, there's a constant truth that spans all generations and people on this planet. The direction in which we focus our thoughts, words, and actions will profoundly affect our quality of life.

Think of it. Words can start wars.

And when used with care and intention, words can help restore peace.

The power of life and death is in the tongue. *We're talking about some pretty incredible power.*

KEY CHAPTER TAKEAWAYS:

- What do we stand for?

- Does what we stand for help others around us to live more fulfilling lives?

- The things we want to be known for will help shape the direction in which we focus our thoughts, words, and actions.

CHAPTER SEVEN: NO APOLOGY? NO ISSUE.

PART 1: Entitlement Weakens Us

It can be strangely satisfying to hold on to emotional offenses. In fact, after a while, we may even feel we're somewhat of an authority on being on the receiving end of those wrongdoings. Many people even seem to gain a slight sense of significance from this.

There are far better, healthier ways to find significance.

Many times, it's harder to let go of offenses entirely because we feel we're entitled to an apology. *(I mean, there's got to be some sense of justice, right?)*

While that may be true, this is the liberating reality: ***our happiness or ability to move forward in life does not depend on someone else's decision to apologize to us.***

We do NOT need anybody else's permission to stop holding on so tightly to the wrongs and let them go.

I know. It's hard to let go of the tough stuff in life.

But nobody wins when we hold on to hurt or bitterness. In fact, when we hold on to resentment, we're the ones getting harmed in that game.

Think of it – the one who inflicted the toxic words on us might not even realize what they've done! Or maybe they're habitual offenders who still choose not to own their stuff. Unfortunately, this person often leaves a trail of pain and ruination everywhere they go.

In our journey to work through dealing with toxic thoughts, let's remember something important. Let's be careful not to allow

ourselves to sink to the levels from which we're working so hard to overcome.

Friend, you are NOT responsible for the toxic words or actions of others. That's not on you. When you tend to take that burden on, remember you now have filters ready to use. They will help to clarify situations like this too.

PART 2: Forgiving Makes Us Stronger

We are responsible for our own stories, though – they're a work in progress, and they can continually be revised!

I want to encourage you with something that's easy to say, but not as simple to act on.

Freedom from those harmful words is available at the other end of forgiveness.

It's been said that to forgive is a sign of weakness. To be truly strong, one must hold tight unswervingly to personal vendettas, striking back when the opportunity avails itself.

But nothing could be further from the truth! In reality, forgiving someone is one of the most powerful, freeing actions we can take.

Here's why.

Remember that earlier reference to the soundtrack of negative words that replay in our minds? You may know it better as another description, 'rumination,' meaning thoughts keep being pondered, meditated on, or rehearsed repeatedly.

Choosing to forgive cuts the power from that rumination track.

Forgiveness causes that superhighway of negative thought patterns we've carved out in our minds to become less traveled. And highways that are not well used will soon become expendable. In the meantime, as our awareness springs into action, new roadways are forged in our minds, resulting in new thought patterns.

So, if I'm going to rehearse a soundtrack in life, wouldn't it be more effective to spend time reminding myself of the good? Embracing what I stand for, am grateful for, and aim for?

Many of us also believe forgiving means we just become a doormat for someone else, so they can keep walking all over us.

That's not what forgiveness is, friend. That's being taken advantage of and only causes pain.

But we can view those harmful actions through the filter's lens. When we do, this can help us see the situation with improved accuracy.

Consider this for a moment: when we choose to forgive, we're not saying the person did no wrong.

Instead, when we forgive, we are choosing to free ourselves from being stuck under the weight of the situation that person created.

You may be thinking, *"but hold on! If I forgive that person, won't it be the same as me admitting what the other individual did is okay? Like they're off the hook now?"*

You're right – some things people say or do are nearly impossible to fathom. But when we forgive someone, we're not saying *"they're off the hook."*

We don't actually have the personal authority to let someone else off the hook.

But when we choose forgiveness, we are the ones who reap the positive rewards. This action helps us be released from that heavy burden – a weight that was never ours to carry in the first place.

Think about that.

When we choose that action, our perspectives cannot help but shift in positive ways. Releasing those hurtful words, we've held onto can feel like a beacon of light shining brightly near the rocky shores of life, offering us a way forward.

And since we're made up of mind, body, and spirit, we're a package deal. When even one area of our lives is affected, it impacts everything. That means choosing to forgive can actually benefit our physical health in amazing ways too!

After I released the negative words, the heaviness of those former toxic thoughts held less and less influence on my perception.

I forgave the person freely for the words spoken over me that day in my hospital bed. No longer was I stuck beneath the weight of the sender's negativity. In the breath of a prayer, I forgave any additional words spoken by others that had compounded over time as well.

And the gravity of those words lifted. Those words no longer held their original sway over me.

My story began to be rewritten.

KEY CHAPTER TAKEAWAYS:

- **Entitlement Weakens Us** – Our happiness in life is not dependent on someone's ability to apologize to us. When we hold on to grudges or bitterness, it hurts us, not them.

- **Forgiving Makes Us Stronger** – When we forgive, we choose to free ourselves from being stuck from the weight of the situation the other person created.

  ⇒ The weight was never ours to take on to begin with.

  ⇒ We're connected in mind, body, and spirit: when one part of us suffers, it can affect our whole being. Even in the breath of a prayer, we can choose to forgive.

  ⇒ Choosing to forgive cuts the power from the rumination track in our minds.

  ⇒ A choice to forgive allows for new, healthier patterns of thought to be forged in our minds.

CHAPTER EIGHT: HOPE IS AHEAD

The fact that you've stayed with me this far says something. It tells me you're ready to take action for yourself or help someone you care about.

That's so good.

Regardless of complications or challenges, I believe there's a way forward.

When negative words are spoken over us, we have an acute responsibility to ourselves to assess and filter them first through our standard of thought.

It only takes a moment to do, but the results can last a lifetime. Once negative words pass through the filter, we can decide where they need to be directed.

I want to see better days ahead for you. Days where your awareness becomes so crystal-clear with firmly established new habits, that negative thoughts of others can no longer get past your filter.

I envision a more compelling future where you realize just how much potential you really have within you to make a difference in this world.

The world needs YOU and who you're designed to be!

No matter where you've been or how many times you've experienced the pain of destructive words in the past, I'm excited to know that there are tools you can use to move forward.

If you're ready to be released from the weight of past toxicity, I encourage you to filter those words again through those three filters, to see them at last for what they are.

And when you're ready to take your life to the next level, consider the strength of forgiveness. There's no downside to forgiveness – the release YOU will experience from that lifted weight will be YOUR win.

The three filters can help you accelerate the process of shedding those words from our lives for good, clarifying future experiences.

The day you decide to use these filters, you'll start to say "yes" to a healthier mindset – and "no more" to polluting thoughts.

You're choosing a life where you value clean beauty for the mind – where living well begins.

And that one decision has the potential to make a powerful, positive impact on the rest of your life.

KEY CHAPTER TAKEAWAYS:

- Regardless of how many times you've experienced the pain of toxic words, there is hope!

- There are tools you have ready to use, to say *"yes"* to a healthier mindset.

- You no longer need to settle for allowing toxic words to remain in your mind.

CONCLUDING THOUGHTS

The book's title 'Clean Beauty for the Mind' comes from an 'Aha' moment I had.

When the moment happened, I realized it wasn't enough that I felt personally equipped to move forward from negative words, past or present. I felt compelled to share it with you too. I want to help you realize there is no need to settle for less than the potential you've been created for.

If this helps even one person move forward, to me, it will have been so worth it to share today.

I believe that the kind of 'Clean Beauty for the Mind' we've discussed is much more profound than just an absence of pollutants.

Instead, it's a way of being, a standard for living that goes far beyond our most flawless selfie ever could.

The highest form of beauty begins in our minds. The way we take care of our thoughts will determine much of our future.

And if these words have resonated with you in some way, and you're ready to take action to safeguard your future, I want you to know that I'm cheering you on!

Whether you use my filters or establish your own, you need to know that you're making an excellent decision for a better tomorrow.

Equipped with a new perspective, you're ready to choose a significant step forward.

*May you feel empowered to know that you are never helpless —
even when someone tries again to plant seeds of negativity in your
mind, you've got this!*

And if those words have been rooted too long, I hope that a new
awareness has emerged within you too, and you're ready. You're
prepared to re-filter those words a second time and take significant
action.

I believe in you. I know you can take steps every day to prevent
future toxic seeds from gaining ground.

*Imagine a world where everyone chose to take a few moments to
first evaluate words before accepting them blindly or retaliating with
hurt.*

What an incredible difference that would make.

Begin to think about or meditate on what CAN be — on the
potential that awaits in your future, when you take these positive
steps to win.

Set a standard for yourself, for what you choose to allow inside,
and begin to stand on that. But establish it on a solid foundation, so it
works. Then, if you need ideas, lean into the good stuff, the pure,
honest, integral, and lovely.

***These new thoughts can help lead to incredibly clean beauty for
the mind. A place of health and restoration.***

*Remember, choosing to live this way doesn't mean negative words
won't be spoken over us again. Not at all.* In fact, we should anticipate
it because that's part of life!

But there's no need to lose hope in the process.

Instead, we can now face those situations head-on with a new perception, dealing with them instantly with filters we're establishing.

We may not be able to change things for everyone at once – but we can absolutely start with one and build from there.

Change begins with you.

You can do this!

You can start the journey today and help inspire others to do the same.

You, my friend, can even help us begin a movement of hope. A place where clean beauty for the mind becomes an impetus for extraordinary change.

The decision to impact our future for the better is within reach. But it begins with a choice. So, let's choose well.

Even though I may still have a red flag when someone gifts me homemade food to this day, now that I have my filter ready, I'll try it!

BIBLIOGRAPHY

1 Waaal, (no date listed) *Patterns in our Brain*, #Same Here Global Mental Health Movement
https://samehereglobal.org/blog/patterns-in-our-brain

2 Miller, Donald, (January 5, 2022) *Hero on A Mission,* Harper Collins
https://www.goodbooks.io/books/hero-on-a-mission

3 Medically Reviewed by Dan Brennan, MD (February 3, 2022) *What is a Victim Mentality?* Web MD *https://www.webmd.com/mental-health/what-is-a-victim-mentality*

ACKNOWLEDGEMENTS

Thank you to my incredible family for your loving support and encouragement as I keep learning on this amazing journey of life. I adore you, and the uniqueness each of you brings to the world. You truly inspire me to want to keep growing! I'm so grateful that I have the true blessing of calling you "family."

I'm also grateful for wonderful people in my life who so succinctly offered their valuable feedback on the very first draft of this book. I wanted this content to impact and resonate with people in a lasting way, regardless of where they were at in life, so feedback mattered. A big shout-out to these amazing individuals for their great input and encouragement: Bill Markham, Alka McArthur, Beatrice P., Shelley Munnings, and Donna Jo Hewitt.

Speaking of pretty wonderful people, it is also my honour to thank the amazing Laurie Snure for her invaluable help with formatting the various versions of this book. When one first sets out to write, the tendency is to think "Okay, how hard could it really be to format?" (If you're a writer, you're likely laughing quietly to yourself right now at the audacity of the question.) Laurie, thank you for your generosity and for the way you've used your gifts to shine.

I want to thank God for inspiring people to write down powerful, timeless words of encouragement that have echoed through the halls of history within ancient texts. The words still remain timeless, and have impacted me in deep ways in life, offering unmatched clarity and wisdom for today.

Finally, I want to thank ***you,*** valued reader for choosing to pick up this book and reading the words. I've written with you in mind because I believe in you. My sincere hope is that after reading this, those negative words you've lived with for too long will lose their sway in your mind. Life is way too precious a gift to hold on to things that can harm us. I truly DO believe that you can move forward, even through negative situations. Friend, I hope I have the honour of hearing a bit of your story someday too.

ABOUT THE AUTHOR

Karlene Markham has spent her life exploring how to maximize human potential. Whether with her family, business or volunteering, she loves to equip others to embrace new perspectives, and help them reach their goals. Her unique ability to inspire and empower others in various leadership settings has helped to motivate people to this end.

Karlene is married to an amazing guy named Bill, adores spending time with her growing family, loves being outdoors and resides in the beautiful nation of Canada.

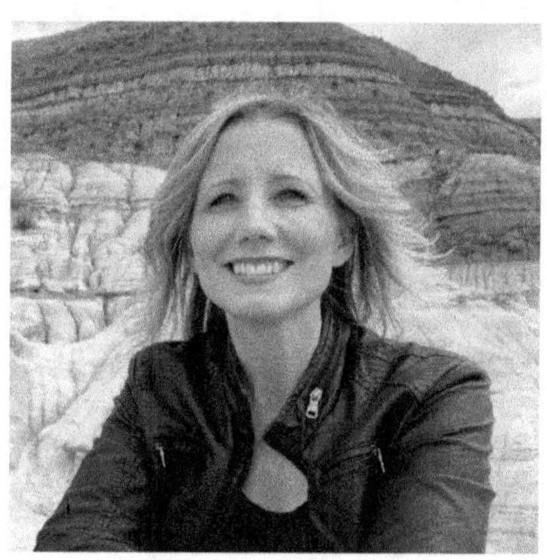

Follow Karlene on...

⇒ Instagram: #cleanbeautyforthemind
⇒ Facebook: @cleanbeautyforthemind

www.cleanbeautyforthemind.com